NAVIGATING THE LANDSCAPE OF PSYCHEDELICS AND DEPRESSION

Table of Contents

INTRODUCTION

A Ray of Hope in the Shadow of Darkness

Imagine a world where the disabling effects of depression lifts, replaced by a ray of hope shining as the potential of psychedelic therapy emerges offering a possibilities to those battling the darkness of depression.

This book we will explore this exciting but complex field of psychedelic therapy as it applies to depression. Lets begin by understanding depression, its grip on daily lives and the limitations of current treatments. We will then look into the history and science of psychedelics, their diverse forms and the many ways they interact with the human brain.

You will read about real stories of transformation will bring to life the profound impact of psychedelic therapy, to show the possibility of hope and renewed with it's therapeutic effects. It will equip you with the necessary knowledge you need to navigate psychedelic therapy responsibly and safely.

The discovery requires open-mindedness and a willingness to challenge the status quo. We'll look into the legal and ethical considerations with transparency in order to demystify the challenges and opportunities ahead. This is not a one cure for all, but a potential therapy with risks and rewards just like any other treatment and must be carefully understood, evaluated and considered.

Ultimately, this book is here to empower you to take full control of your mental well-being. It is paramount that you explore the potential of both psychedelic therapy and other alternative approaches to discover what suits your needs best. It is only through collaborative inquiry and open dialogue, that we can break down established stigma and foster a future where individuals and communities find lasting healing and mental wellness.

If you are ready to step into the this adventure, turn the page, and let's explore the potential of psychedelics use for those struggling with depression.

Part 1: Understanding Depression and the Need for Alternatives

Chapter 1: Defining Depression: Symptoms, Causes, and Treatments

Depression isn't simply feeling blue or down for a short period. It's a persistent sadness and darkness that engulfs over your life, robbing you of joy, motivation, and hope. It's a never ending and constant voice that is whispering negativity, isolating you from the world, and leaving you feeling trapped. Understanding the depths and complexities of depression is crucial in order to navigate, and seek help.

Unveiling the Symptoms:

The symptoms of depression vary from person to person, but some common signs include:

- Persistent sadness or emptiness: This deep sadness isn't just temporary moodiness; it lingers and permeates your daily life.
- Loss of interest or pleasure in activities you once enjoyed: Whether it's hobbies, work, or spending time with loved ones, the things that used to bring you joy become devoid of it.
- Changes in appetite or weight: Some people experience significant weight loss due to decreased appetite, while others experience weight gain due to emotional eating.
- Trouble sleeping or sleeping too much: Sleep disturbances are hallmark symptoms of depression, ranging from insomnia and waking up early to excessive sleepiness.
- Loss of energy or fatigue: Feeling constantly drained and lacking the motivation to complete daily tasks.

- Feelings of worthlessness or guilt: This can manifest as self-criticism, blaming yourself for everything, and believing you're not good enough.
- Difficulty thinking, concentrating, or making decisions: This can cloud your thoughts, make it hard to focus, and hinder your ability to make everyday choices.
- Increased restlessness or agitation: Some people experience physical restlessness, pacing, or fidgeting, while others feel mentally agitated and irritable.
- Recurrent thoughts of death or suicide: While not everyone with depression has suicidal thoughts, it's crucial to consider these as serious warnings and seek help immediately.
- Understanding the Causes:

The causes of depression are complex and vary between individuals. While there's no single answer, some contributing factors include:

- Biological factors: Brain chemistry imbalances, particularly involving serotonin and dopamine, can play a role.
- Genetics: Having a family history of depression increases your risk.
- Medical conditions: Chronic illnesses, thyroid problems, and chronic pain can trigger depression.
- Life stressors: Traumatic events, loss, financial difficulties, and relationship problems can be major triggers.
- Personality traits: Perfectionism, negative thinking patterns, and low self-esteem can make you more vulnerable.

Exploring the Treatments:

While depression can be overwhelming, remember there is hope and treatments that can help you manage symptoms and reclaim your life.

Some of the key options that can help you manage depression are:

- Medication: Antidepressants can help regulate brain chemistry and alleviate symptoms. Different types work for different people, so finding the right medication may require trial and error.
- Therapy: Talk therapy, like cognitive-behavioural therapy (CBT), can help you identify and change negative thinking patterns, develop coping skills, and improve relationships.
- Electroconvulsive therapy (ECT): This treatment involves sending electrical currents to the brain and is typically used for severe depression when other options haven't been effective.
- Lifestyle changes: Exercise, healthy eating, regular sleep, and reducing stress can significantly improve your mood and overall well-being.
- Complementary and alternative therapies: While not a substitute for traditional treatment, options like mindfulness meditation, yoga, and acupuncture can provide additional support.

Finding Your Path:

Remember, there's no one-size-fits-all approach to overcoming depression. It's crucial to work with a healthcare professional to develop a personalized treatment plan that addresses your specific needs and circumstances. Be patient, don't hesitate to seek help, and trust that you can find the tools and resources to navigate this challenging journey.

Chapter 2: The Limitations of Traditional Treatment and Why We Need New Solutions to treat depression

While traditional treatments like medication and therapy have offered solace and relief to millions grappling with depression, their limitations persist. This chapter delves into these limitations, highlighting the need for exploring new avenues, including the potential of psychedelics therapy.

The Ray of Hope:

Traditional treatments are the first line of defence against depression, and for many, they provide life-changing results. Antidepressants help regulate brain chemistry, while therapy equips individuals with tools to address negative thought patterns and develop coping mechanisms. However, it's crucial to acknowledge that they aren't perfect solutions for everyone.

Unveiling the Shadows:

Here are some key limitations of traditional treatments of depression:

- Limited Effectiveness: Not everyone responds well to medication, and finding the right combination can be a lengthy and frustrating process. Some people experience debilitating side effects like fatigue, sexual dysfunction, and emotional blunting.
- Accessibility Barriers: Cost, lack of insurance coverage, and limited access to qualified mental health professionals create significant barriers for many, particularly in underserved communities.

- Relapse Rates: Even with successful treatment, depression can return, leaving individuals feeling discouraged and vulnerable. Existing treatments may not effectively prevent future episodes.
- Addressing the Root Causes: While managing symptoms is crucial, traditional treatments may not adequately address the underlying causes of depression, such as early life trauma, chronic stress, or social inequalities.

The Call for Innovation:

These limitations highlight the urgent need for exploring new approaches to combating depression. We need novel therapeutic options that are:

- More effective: Targeting a wider range of depression presentations and offering lasting relief for those who don't respond well to existing treatments.
- More accessible: Overcoming cost and access barriers to ensure everyone has the opportunity to access effective treatment.
- Focusing on prevention: Developing strategies to prevent the onset of depression, especially in at-risk populations.
- Addressing root causes: Moving beyond symptom management to delve into and address the underlying factors contributing to depression.

Enter the Frontier: Psychedelics as a Potential Answer?

In recent years, research on psychedelics has reemerged, presenting a glimmer of hope in the fight against depression. While this field is still in its early stages, preliminary findings suggest their potential to address some of the limitations mentioned above. In the next chapter, we'll delve deeper into the world of psychedelics, exploring their mechanisms of action and the promising results emerging from ongoing research.

Important Note:

This chapter does not intend to diminish the value of traditional treatments. They remain crucial resources for many individuals with depression. However, acknowledging their limitations and the need for further innovation is essential for advancing mental healthcare and offering improved solutions for those struggling.

Stay tuned as we embark on a journey into the intriguing world of psychedelics and their potential role in overcoming depression.

Chapter 3: Beyond Medication: Exploring Alternative Approaches to Mental Wellness

While medication and therapy form the backbone of traditional depression treatment, a holistic approach recognizes the power of venturing beyond the medicine cabinet. This chapter explores complementary and alternative approaches that can empower you to proactively manage your mental well-being and support traditional treatment options.

Embracing a Holistic Perspective:

Mental health isn't just about medication. It encompasses the intricate interplay of your physical, emotional, and social aspects. By cultivating a holistic approach, you address depression on multiple levels, creating a foundation for lasting well-being.

Lifestyle Tweaks for a Brighter Mindset:

Our day-to-day choices significantly impact our mood and resilience. Consider incorporating these lifestyle changes:

* Nourishing your body: Choose whole, unprocessed foods rich in nutrients that support brain function and overall health. Stay hydrated, and avoid excessive sugar and caffeine.
* Moving your body: Regular physical activity, even moderate-intensity exercises like brisk walking, releases endorphins, natural mood boosters, and reduces stress. Find activities you enjoy to stay motivated.
* Prioritizing sleep: Aim for 7-8 hours of quality sleep each night. Establish a consistent sleep schedule, create a relaxing bedtime routine, and avoid screens before bed.

- Mindfulness and meditation: These practices train your mind to be present and non-judgmental, reducing stress, anxiety, and negative thought patterns. Explore various techniques and find what resonates with you.
- Connecting with nature: Spending time outdoors in natural environments has proven benefits for reducing stress, enhancing mood, and promoting overall well-being.
- Nurturing social connections: Strong social bonds provide support, love, and a sense of belonging, fostering resilience against depression. Spend time with loved ones, join social groups, or volunteer in your community.

Complementary and Alternative Therapies:

These therapies can serve as complementary tools alongside traditional treatment, not a replacement:

- **Yoga and Tai Chi**: These mind-body practices combine physical postures with breathing exercises, promoting relaxation, reducing stress, and improving mindfulness.

- **Acupuncture**: This traditional Chinese medicine technique involves inserting thin needles into specific points on the body, aiming to restore balance and improve energy flow.

- **Massage therapy**: Physical touch can reduce stress, anxiety, and muscle tension, contributing to relaxation and well-being.

- **Art therapy**: Expressing emotions and experiences through creative activities can be cathartic and insightful, fostering emotional processing and self-discovery.

Remember: Consult your healthcare professional before starting any new therapy to ensure it's safe and suitable for you.

Empowering Yourself:

Beyond specific techniques, remember:

* Knowledge is power: Educate yourself about depression, its triggers, and available treatment options.

* Self-compassion is key: Be kind and understanding towards yourself. Depression doesn't define you.

* Celebrate small victories: Track your progress, acknowledge your efforts, and celebrate even small steps forward.

* Advocacy matters: Raise awareness about mental health, advocate for better access to resources, and challenge stigma surrounding depression.

Combining Forces:

Remember, this chapter doesn't advocate for abandoning traditional treatment. When combined with a holistic approach that includes lifestyle changes, complementary therapies, and a supportive network, medication and therapy can be even more effective.

By exploring these alternative approaches, you empower yourself to actively participate in your healing journey and build lasting resilience against depression. In the next chapter, we'll delve into a particularly intriguing frontier: the potential of psychedelics for treating depression.

Part 2: Unveiling the World of Psychedelics

Chapter 4: A Historical Journey: From Ancient Rituals to Modern Research

Step into the psychedelic frontier, a world where ancient wisdom meets modern science in a quest to unlock new avenues for healing. This chapter embarks on a fascinating historical journey, tracing the use of psychedelics from their ritualistic origins to their controversial ban and the recent resurgence of research with a focus on depression.

From Shamans to Science:

Our story begins millennia ago, where psychedelic substances like psilocybin (magic mushrooms) and ayahuasca were woven into the fabric of ancient cultures. They were used for spiritual ceremonies, divination, and healing practices, fostering profound experiences and insights into the self and the world.

The Age of Exploration:

As civilizations expanded, encounters with these substances continued. From indigenous tribes in the Americas to mystics in the Middle East, psychedelics remained a potent force in diverse cultures. However, the focus shifted from ritualistic practices to individual exploration and self-discovery.

The Psychedelic Boom:

In the mid-20th century, a cultural revolution sparked renewed interest in psychedelics. Pioneers like Aldous Huxley and Timothy Leary explored their mind-expanding potential, leading to widespread experimentation and research. However, concerns about misuse and potential dangers led to their prohibition in many countries.

A Decade of Darkness:

The 1970s and 80s marked a period of dormancy for psychedelic research. Stigma, legal restrictions, and methodological challenges hindered exploration. However, the underground community continued to use psychedelics for personal growth and spiritual exploration, keeping the flame alive.

The Dawn of a New Era:

Since the turn of the millennium, a renaissance in psychedelic research has emerged. Scientists, no longer driven by the counterculture movement, are conducting rigorous studies with strict ethical guidelines and safety protocols. This renewed interest is fueled by:

Improved understanding of the brain: Advanced imaging techniques and neuroscientific research provide insights into how psychedelics impact brain function and neural pathways.
Shifting societal perspectives: Growing openness to alternative approaches to mental health and increased recognition of the limitations of traditional treatments create fertile ground for exploration.
Promising preliminary results: Early studies suggest that psychedelics may be effective in treating depression, anxiety,

addiction, and other mental health conditions, warranting further investigation.

A Look Ahead:

While the future of psychedelic research remains uncertain, the historical journey offers valuable lessons. By acknowledging the past, respecting traditional knowledge, and conducting responsible research, we can unlock the potential of these substances to offer new hope for those struggling with mental health challenges.
Stay tuned as we delve deeper into the science behind psychedelics and their potential role in treating depression in the next chapter.

Chapter 5: Unveiling the Mechanisms: How Psychedelics Impact the Brain and Depression

While the visual distortions and altered states of consciousness associated with psychedelics may capture the public imagination, their potential role in treating depression rests on a far deeper level. This chapter delves into the science behind the scenes, exploring how these substances interact with the brain and offer a glimmer of hope for those struggling with this debilitating condition.

Beyond the Sensory Spectacle:

Imagine your brain as a vast network of interconnected pathways, constantly firing and shaping your thoughts, emotions, and experiences. Depression often results from rigid, unhealthy patterns established within these pathways. Enter psychedelics, which seemingly possess the unique ability to loosen the grip of these patterns, fostering new connections and perspectives.

Unlocking Neuroplasticity's Potential:

One key mechanism lies in neuroplasticity, the brain's remarkable ability to change and adapt. Traditional treatments like antidepressants can nudge this process, but psychedelics appear to act as turbochargers. Studies suggest they increase the growth of new connections and enhance the flexibility of existing ones, paving the way for new ways of thinking, feeling, and responding to the world. This newfound plasticity might be crucial for breaking free from the negative thought cycles that fuel depression.

Rewiring Emotional Responses:

Depression often involves a struggle to acknowledge and process difficult emotions. Psychedelics, however, hold promise in facilitating this process. Research suggests they enhance emotional processing, allowing individuals to confront and reframe negative emotions that contribute to their depressive state. By providing a safe space for exploration and acceptance, these substances might pave the way for emotional healing and growth.

Quieting the Inner Critic:

Have you ever been stuck in a loop of negative self-talk? The Default Mode Network (DMN) plays a key role in this internal critique. This network, when overactive, can lead to rumination and self-criticism, further deepening the depressive state. Interestingly, studies suggest that psychedelics can temporarily quiet the DMN, offering individuals a respite from their inner critic and opening the door to new perspectives and self-compassion.

The Chemical Orchestra:

Our mood and emotions are largely governed by an intricate dance of neurotransmitters, chemical messengers in the brain. Among these, serotonin plays a critical role in regulating mood and happiness. While traditional antidepressants aim to boost serotonin levels, psychedelics interact with its receptors in unique ways, potentially leading to more nuanced and long-lasting changes. Additionally, they influence other neurotransmitters involved in mood regulation, further shaping the complex interplay that affects our mental well-being.

Exploring the Psychedelic Spectrum:

- Psilocybin and MDMA stand out as the most researched psychedelics for depression treatment, but the frontier extends beyond them:

- LSD: Early data suggests its potential in reducing depression symptoms by enhancing emotional processing.

- Ayahuasca: This traditional brew containing DMT shows promise in anecdotal reports, but large-scale studies are needed to confirm its effectiveness and safety.

- Ketamine: Already approved for treatment-resistant depression, its rapid-acting effect offers a novel approach, though its exact mechanism remains under investigation.

A Word of Caution:

Despite the encouraging findings, it's crucial to acknowledge the limitations and cautionary notes:

Research in its early stages: While early results are promising, more large-scale, long-term studies are needed to solidify the scientific understanding and confirm the efficacy and safety of psychedelic therapy for depression.

Individualized responses: Just like medication, psychedelics don't work the same for everyone. Set, setting, and individual differences play a significant role in shaping the experience and outcome.

Potential risks and limitations: Psychedelic experiences can be challenging and unpredictable, even in controlled settings. Professional guidance and careful screening are essential to ensure safety and maximize potential benefits.

Unlocking Hope:

Understanding the mechanisms by which psychedelics interact with the brain offers a tantalizing glimpse into their potential for treating depression. However, the science alone doesn't paint the full picture. In the next chapter, we'll dive deeper by exploring the lived experiences of individuals who have found hope and healing through psychedelic therapy for depression. Their stories will offer a personal dimension to this emerging field, highlighting the potential impact on real lives.

Stay tuned as we embark on a journey through personal narratives and uncover the transformative power of these substances for those battling depression.

Chapter 6: A Spectrum of Options: Exploring Different Psychedelic Therapies

As we journey deeper into the psychedelic frontier, it's important to recognize that no single substance holds the universal key to unlocking healing from depression. Instead, a spectrum of options exists, each with its unique characteristics, potential benefits, and considerations. In this chapter, we'll embark on a guided exploration of the leading contenders in the realm of psychedelic-assisted therapy for depression:

1. Psilocybin:

The Magic Mushroom: Derived from certain species of mushrooms, psilocybin is currently the most researched psychedelic for depression. Early studies show promising results in reducing symptoms, potentially by enhancing neuroplasticity and emotional processing.

Treatment Protocol: Typically administered in 2-3 sessions, with careful preparation, support, and integration practices.

Considerations: Requires a comfortable, controlled setting and experienced guides. Not currently legal for therapeutic use in most countries.

2. MDMA (Ecstasy):

The Love Drug: MDMA, known for its social and emotional connection-enhancing effects, is being investigated for its potential to address trauma-related depression. It may facilitate emotional processing and foster self-compassion.

Treatment Protocol: Similar to psilocybin, MDMA therapy involves carefully guided sessions with emotional support and integration practices.

Considerations: Rigorous screening for potential contraindications is crucial. MDMA remains a Schedule I controlled substance in most countries, limiting research and accessibility.

3. LSD:

The Mind Expander: While historically associated with counterculture movements, LSD is regaining research interest for its potential in treating depression, possibly by promoting cognitive flexibility and emotional insight.

Treatment Protocol: Limited research at this stage, making protocols less defined compared to psilocybin and MDMA.

Considerations: Due to its potent nature and potential for adverse reactions, careful screening and experienced guides are essential. Legal restrictions hinder research and therapeutic use in many regions.

4. Ketamine:

The Anesthetic: Already approved for treatment-resistant depression, Ketamine works differently than classical psychedelics, offering rapid-acting relief through mechanisms still being unraveled.
Treatment Protocol: Typically administered in low doses through nasal spray or infusion, requiring close monitoring by healthcare professionals.

Considerations: While effective for some, ketamine's long-term effects and potential risks require further investigation. Limited availability and potential for misuse raise concerns.

5. Ayahuasca:

The Shamanic Brew: This traditional Amazonian brew containing DMT shows anecdotal promise in treating depression but lacks rigorous scientific evaluation. Its complex pharmacology and intense cultural context necessitate extreme caution and responsible exploration.

Considerations: Legal restrictions and potential risks associated with its complex composition and strong effects demand careful consideration and responsible guidance.

Remember: This is not an exhaustive list, and the psychedelic landscape is constantly evolving. Choosing the "right" option requires careful research, individual needs assessment, and guidance from qualified healthcare professionals familiar with this emerging field.

Beyond the Substances:

- It's crucial to remember that psychedelic therapy is more than just the substances themselves. Each treatment program emphasizes:

- Set and Setting: Creating a safe, supportive environment with experienced guides is vital for a positive and therapeutic experience.

- Preparation and Education: Understanding the process, potential challenges, and expectations is crucial for informed participation.

- Integration: Processing insights and experiences gained during the sessions is essential for lasting positive outcomes.

Exploring the Spectrum:

As we explore this new frontier, embracing openness, responsible inquiry, and respect for individual experiences is key. By understanding the spectrum of options, their potential benefits, and limitations, we can navigate this emerging field with a sense of informed hope and caution. In the next chapter, we'll delve into the transformative power of these therapies through the captivating stories of individuals who have found healing through psychedelic experiences.

Stay tuned as we witness the impact of these substances on real lives and explore the potential for a brighter future for those struggling with depression.

Part 3: Exploring Psychedelic Therapy: Risks, Benefits, and Practicalities

Chapter 7: Real Stories of Transformation: Personal Accounts of Healing with Psychedelics

We've delved into the history, science, and diverse options within the psychedelic frontier. Now, it's time to shift our focus to the most powerful testament to the potential of this emerging field: the transformative stories of individuals who have found healing from depression through psychedelic therapy.

Beyond the Statistics:

While promising research findings paint a hopeful picture, statistics alone can't convey the profound impact these experiences can have on real lives. In this chapter, we'll meet individuals who have bravely shared their personal journeys. Through their voices, we'll witness the struggles, uncertainties, and ultimately, the transformative power of psychedelic therapy.

A Tapestry of Voices:

Sarah: Struggling with treatment-resistant depression for years, Sarah found relief and a renewed sense of self-compassion through psilocybin therapy.
David: Haunted by childhood trauma and crippling anxiety, David experienced emotional breakthroughs and a newfound connection to life through MDMA- assisted therapy.

Maria: After losing her husband, Maria grappled with debilitating grief. Ayahuasca, steeped in tradition and guided by indigenous healers, led her on a path of acceptance and healing.

Each Journey Unique:

Every story is unique, reflecting the diverse experiences and needs of individuals. Some journeys might be filled with intense emotions, while others unfold with quiet introspection. However, a common thread emerges: a profound shift in perspective, a renewed sense of hope, and an empowered approach to healing.

Beyond the Hype:

It's crucial to acknowledge that psychedelic therapy is not a magical cure-all. It's a challenging and demanding process, requiring preparation, commitment, and support. Individual responses vary, and setbacks or integration difficulties can occur.

Hope with Responsibility:

These stories offer a ray of hope, but caution is vital. Remember, this field is young, and extensive research and ethical considerations are essential. Approaching this path with informed consent, responsible sourcing, and guidance from qualified healthcare professionals is paramount.

Beyond the Individual:

The personal transformations we witness in these stories also highlight the potential societal impact of this emerging field. By offering a new, evidence-based approach to mental health, psychedelics have the potential to:

- Reduce the burden of depression and other mental health challenges
- Challenge stigma and promote open dialogue about mental health
- Empower individuals to take ownership of their healing journeys

Chapter 8: Setting the Stage: Ensuring Safe and Responsible Psychedelic Experiences

The potential of psychedelics for treating depression is sparking hope, but venturing into this uncharted territory demands informed and responsible action. Before embarking on a psychedelic journey, understanding the crucial elements for safety, ethical considerations, and maximizing potential benefits is paramount.

Building on Solid Ground:

Responsible psychedelic experiences rest on four foundational pillars:

Set: Your mental and emotional preparation is crucial. Entering with a clear intention, addressing fears and expectations, and ensuring emotional stability are essential.

Setting: The physical and social environment plays a vital role. Choose a safe, comfortable space free from distractions, with trusted guides or facilitators present.

Substance: Understanding the specific substance, its potential effects, and potential risks is vital. Research thoroughly and choose reputable sources.

Support: Access to qualified professionals experienced in guiding psychedelic journeys and providing ongoing support throughout the process is crucial.

Beyond the Basic Principles:

Ethical considerations and responsible sourcing are equally important:

- Informed Consent: Ensure you fully understand the potential benefits and risks before participating in any psychedelic experience.

- Responsible Sourcing: Avoid illegal or unregulated substances to ensure purity and minimize risks. Seek ethical, legal sources, if available.

- Cultural Respect: Approach traditional practices with respect and avoid cultural appropriation. Seek guidance from experienced practitioners within those traditions.

- Harm Reduction: Integrate harm reduction practices to minimize potential risks, such as setting clear boundaries, avoiding mixing substances, and prioritizing mental and emotional well-being.

Beyond the Individual:

Responsible action extends beyond the personal experience:

- Advocacy: Support organizations advocating for responsible research, safe access, and destigmatization of psychedelic therapies.

- Community Building: Connect with communities exploring psychedelics responsibly and ethically, fostering learning and support.

- Critical Thinking: Approach all information, including personal accounts, with a critical eye. Seek verified sources and engage in responsible discourse.

Remember:

- Psychedelics are powerful substances and can be unpredictable. Treat them with respect and caution.
- There is no guaranteed outcome, and individual experiences vary greatly.
- The path to healing is often complex and multifaceted. Psychedelics may be a valuable tool, but they are not a singular solution.
- Seek professional guidance and support throughout your journey.
- Setting the stage for a safe, responsible, and potentially transformative psychedelic experience requires mindful preparation, informed consent, and ethical considerations. By taking these steps, we can contribute to building a brighter future for mental health and the responsible exploration of this promising frontier.

Chapter 9: Beyond the Trip: The Importance of Integration and Therapy

The psychedelic experience can be profound, opening doors to new perspectives and emotional breakthroughs. But the journey doesn't end with the "trip." Integration, the process of processing and translating your insights into lasting change, is where the real magic happens.

From Peak to Grounding:

Imagine climbing a mountain. Reaching the summit, you witness breathtaking views and gain new insights. However, the truc benefit lies in descending safely and integrating those insights into your everyday life. Similarly, psychedelic experiences offer an ascent to new mental landscapes, but the true transformation unfolds in the valleys of integration.

Why Integration Matters:

- Making sense of the experience: Psychedelic journeys can be intense and symbolically rich. Integration helps you unpack your experiences, understand their meaning, and identify key learnings.
- Embracing lasting change: Without integration, the insights gained during the trip can fade like fleeting dreams. Integration helps you anchor these insights into your daily life and translate them into concrete actions.
- Addressing emotional challenges: Psychedelic experiences can surface difficult emotions. Integration provides a safe space to process these emotions, develop coping mechanisms, and cultivate emotional resilience.

- Preventing post-trip challenges: Integration can help mitigate potential difficulties like confusion, anxiety, or integration crisis, ensuring a smoother transition back to everyday life.

The Tools of Integration:

Remember, integration is a personal and creative process. Different approaches work for different individuals. Here are some options to explore:

- Therapy: Working with a therapist experienced in psychedelic integration can provide invaluable support and guidance as you navigate your experience.
- Journaling: Regularly reflecting on your thoughts, feelings, and insights gained during the trip can help solidify your learning and track your progress.
- Creative expression: Art, music, movement, and other creative outlets can offer powerful ways to process and express your experience.
- Community support: Connecting with others who have had psychedelic experiences can foster understanding, connection, and shared learning.
- Meditation and mindfulness practices: Cultivating present-moment awareness can help you integrate your new perspectives and navigate challenging emotions.
- Integration is not a linear process. It may involve revisiting certain themes, encountering setbacks, and experiencing moments of clarity. Remember, be patient with yourself and seek support when needed.

Therapy as a Key Partner:

While various tools can support integration, therapy specifically focused on psychedelic experiences offers unique benefits:

- Safe and confidential space: A therapist provides a safe, non-judgmental space to explore your experience openly and honestly.
- Professional expertise: Therapists trained in psychedelic integration understand the complexities of these experiences and can guide you effectively.
- Addressing past baggage: Childhood trauma, unresolved conflicts, and past experiences can influence your psychedelic journey. Therapy can help address these underlying issues and promote deeper healing.
- Developing coping mechanisms: Therapy can equip you with tools and strategies to manage difficult emotions, navigate life challenges, and sustain positive changes.

Finding the Right Therapist:

When seeking a therapist for psychedelic integration, consider:

- Experience: Look for therapists trained and experienced in psychedelic integration specifically.
- Approach: Explore different therapeutic modalities to find one that resonates with you.
- Personal connection: Feeling comfortable and safe with your therapist is crucial for fostering open communication and trust.

Conclusion:

The psychedelic journey is a powerful catalyst for change, but true transformation unfolds in the fertile ground of integration. By embracing integration and seeking professional support, you can translate your insights into lasting positive change, cultivate emotional well-being, and embark on a brighter path in your life.

Chapter 10: Legal Landscape: Understanding the Regulations and Accessibility

As the potential of psychedelics for treating depression gains traction, navigating the complex legal landscape surrounding their use remains crucial. This chapter delves into the current state of regulations, accessibility, and potential future developments.

A Patchwork Quilt of Laws:

The legal status of psychedelics varies widely across the globe, creating a patchwork quilt of regulations:

- Schedule I: In many countries, including the United States, most psychedelics are classified as Schedule I substances, meaning they have high potential for abuse and no currently accepted medical use. This significantly restricts research and accessibility.
- Decriminalization: Some regions have decriminalized the possession and use of certain substances, like psilocybin in Oregon, though this doesn't equate to legal use for medical purposes.
- Medical Exemptions: A few countries, like Canada, allow medical exemptions for compassionate access to specific psychedelics for individuals with treatment-resistant conditions.
- Research Exemptions: Research exemptions allow controlled studies exploring the therapeutic potential of psychedelics, but these often face bureaucratic hurdles and funding limitations.

Accessibility Challenges:

The legal restrictions translate into accessibility challenges:

- Limited Clinical Trials: Limited research funding and complex regulatory processes hinder the progress of clinical trials, delaying access to potential treatments.
- High Costs: Even in countries with legal exemptions, the high costs associated with therapy and potential legal risks can make it inaccessible for many.
- Lack of Qualified Providers: The limited number of healthcare professionals trained in psychedelic therapy further restricts access.

The Winds of Change:

Despite the challenges, a shift in public perception and legal landscape is underway:

- Growing Public Support: Public opinion polls indicate increasing support for exploring the therapeutic potential of psychedelics.
- Policy Reforms: Decriminalization efforts and growing research interest are pushing for policy reforms and regulatory changes.
- Increased Funding: Increased funding for research and pilot programs offer a glimmer of hope for wider accessibility.

Looking Ahead:

Predicting the future of psychedelic therapy regulations is complex:
- Potential for Continued Progress: Continued research, advocacy, and public support could pave the way for decriminalization, increased research funding, and eventually, wider legal access for therapeutic use.
- Challenges Remain: Legal and ethical considerations, concerns about potential misuse, and the need for robust regulatory frameworks will continue to shape the landscape.

Individual Responsibility:

While the legal landscape evolves, remember:
- Current Regulations: Adhering to existing laws and regulations is crucial to avoid legal consequences.
- Research and Advocacy: Stay informed about ongoing research and advocacy efforts to support responsible exploration and potential policy changes.
- Seek Professional Guidance: If considering psychedelic therapy, prioritize your safety and well-being by working with qualified and legally authorized professionals.

Conclusion:

The legal landscape surrounding psychedelics is complex and constantly evolving. While navigating this landscape requires caution and adherence to current regulations, the potential benefits for treating depression and other mental health conditions warrant continued research, advocacy, and responsible exploration. By staying informed and engaged, we can contribute to a future where safe and effective psychedelic therapies are accessible to those who need them most.

Chapter 11: Addressing the Critics: Ethical Considerations and Potential Risks

As the potential of psychedelics for treating depression sparks excitement, it's essential to acknowledge the ethical considerations and potential risks associated with this emerging field. Open and responsible dialogue addressing these concerns is crucial for navigating this frontier ethically and ensuring it benefits individuals and society as a whole.

Ethical Considerations:

- Informed Consent: Ensuring individuals seeking psychedelic therapy fully understand the potential benefits, risks, and uncertainties involved is paramount.
- Cultural Sensitivity: Respecting cultural context and avoiding exploitation of indigenous practices and knowledge is essential.
- Vulnerable Populations: Protecting vulnerable populations, such as those with pre-existing mental health conditions or undergoing major life changes, requires careful screening and additional safeguards.
- Commercialization: Balancing potential financial benefits with ethical considerations related to accessibility and exploitation is crucial.
- Misinformation and Hype: Countering misinformation and exaggerated claims, while advocating for responsible research and evidence-based approaches, is vital.

Potential Risks:

- Adverse Psychological Reactions: While rare, intense emotions, anxiety, or challenging emotional experiences can occur during psychedelic journeys.
- Psychosis or HPPD: Though uncommon, there's a small risk of triggering or exacerbating pre-existing psychotic conditions or inducing Hallucinogen Persisting Perception Disorder (HPPD).
- Addiction: Although not addictive in the traditional sense, some individuals might develop psychological dependence or misuse patterns.
- Legal Risks: Using psychedelics outside of legal and authorized settings carries legal consequences and safety concerns.

Balancing Hope and Caution:

Despite these considerations, acknowledging the potential risks shouldn't overshadow the glimmer of hope offered by this field. By taking a balanced approach that embraces transparency, prioritizes safety, and addresses ethical concerns, we can maximize the potential for positive outcomes while minimizing risks.

Moving Forward Responsibly:

- Support Rigorous Research: Advocate for and participate in well-designed, ethically sound research initiatives.
- Choose Qualified Providers: Seek guidance from licensed and experienced professionals trained in psychedelic therapy.
- Prioritize Safety: Adhere to legal regulations and prioritize your physical and emotional well-being throughout the process.
- Engage in Open Dialogue: Share your experiences responsibly, challenge misinformation, and contribute to fostering informed public discourse.

Conclusion:

The path forward with psychedelics requires acknowledging both the potential benefits and potential risks. By prioritizing ethical considerations, advocating for responsible research and regulations, and engaging in open dialogue, we can cultivate a future where this promising field contributes to healing and well-being, ensuring its benefits reach those who need them most.

Part 4: Looking Ahead: The Future of Psychedelics and Mental Wellness

Chapter 12: Decoding Your Inner Universe: How Genes Dance with Psychedelics

Imagine entering a vibrant dreamscape, where colours pulse with cosmic intensity and your thoughts take flight like butterflies on the wind. This, my friends, is the potential magic of a psychedelic journey. But have you ever wondered why some people dance with euphoria while others face emotional whirlwinds? The answer, dear reader, lies within the swirling code of your very own DNA.

Yes, that's right! Your genes, those microscopic instruction manuals, subtly influence how you respond to psychedelics. It's like having a personalized soundtrack playing in the background of your trip, influencing the melody and rhythm of your experience.

Before you start envisioning yourself as a walking lab report, remember this: genetics are just one piece of the puzzle. Your environment, upbringing, mindset, and even the type of psychedelic used all play a role. But understanding how your genes might whisper to your trip can be empowering and insightful.

So, let's explore some of the key factors in the gene-psychedelic dance:

1. **Serotonin Symphony:** Picture serotonin as the conductor of your brain's orchestra. Many psychedelics, like psilocybin and LSD, interact with serotonin receptors, influencing mood, perception, and emotional processing. Genes like HTR2A and 5HTTLPR influence how efficiently your brain produces and utilizes serotonin, potentially impacting the intensity and nature of your psychedelic experience.

2. **The Dopamine Dervishes:** Remember that euphoric rush you get from a delicious meal or a thrilling accomplishment? That's dopamine, another key player in the brain's reward system. Certain genes, like COMT and DRD2, affect how your brain handles dopamine, which could influence the degree of pleasure or emotional connection you experience during a psychedelic journey.

3. **The Metabolic Maze:** How your body processes and eliminates psychedelics can also be influenced by genetics. Variations in genes like CYP2D6 and ABCB1 can affect your metabolism, potentially influencing the duration and intensity of your experience.

4. **The Brain's Wiring:** Just like the intricate cables powering a computer, your brain's neural connections influence how information flows and emotions are generated. Genes like BDNF and CACNA1C play a role in this intricate wiring, and some studies suggest they might influence how receptive your brain is to the transformative potential of psychedelics.

Depression's Shadow and the Genetic Dance:

Now, how does this all connect to the dark cloud of depression? Well, research suggests that some of the same genes mentioned above have also been linked to depression susceptibility. This highlights the intricate dance between our genetic makeup and mental health. Understanding how your genes interact with psychedelics might offer valuable insights into their potential effectiveness in alleviating depression symptoms, tailoring treatment approaches, and minimizing potential risks.

But remember, my friend, genetics are not destiny! They simply offer a fascinating glimpse into the potential for personalized psychedelic experiences. The true magic lies within your own unique journey, your willingness to explore, and your commitment to healing.

This is just the beginning of an exciting exploration! As research continues to unravel the intricate tapestry of genes and psychedelics, we'll gain deeper understanding of their personalized effects and potential for mental health breakthroughs. So, embrace your unique genetic symphony, approach your psychedelic journey with respect and mindfulness, and remember: the key to unlocking your inner universe lies not just in your genes, but also in the courageous steps you take on your path to healing.

Disclaimer: This information is for educational purposes only and should not be construed as medical advice. Please consult with a qualified healthcare professional before embarking on any psychedelic journey.

Chapter 13: The Future of Psychedelic Therapy: Ongoing Research and Emerging Trends

As we stand at the threshold of a new era in mental health treatment, the future of psychedelic therapy holds immense promise. This chapter delves into the exciting research advancements, emerging trends, and potential challenges shaping this rapidly evolving field.

The Research Landscape:

The number of research studies exploring the therapeutic potential of psychedelics is exploding. Key areas of investigation include:

- **Mechanism of Action:** Unravelling the complex ways psychedelics interact with the brain to unlock healing and positive change.
- **Treatment Optimization:** Refining protocols, combining psychedelics with other therapies, and exploring different dosing strategies for various conditions.
- **Personalized Medicine:** Tailoring psychedelic therapy to individual needs and genetic predispositions for enhanced efficacy and reduced risks.
- **Expanded Awareness:** Investigating the effectiveness of psychedelics beyond depression to treat anxiety, addiction, PTSD, and other mental health conditions.

Beyond Traditional Psychedelics:

The research landscape extends beyond classic psychedelics like psilocybin and MDMA:

- **Microdosing:** Exploring the potential of low-dose, regular psychedelic use for enhancing creativity, well-being, and cognitive function.
- **Ibogaine:** Investigating the unique properties of this naturally occurring psychedelic in treating addiction and promoting spiritual growth.
- **Ketamine-Assisted Therapy** (KAT): Further refining the use of ketamine, already approved for treatment-resistant depression, and exploring its potential for other conditions.

Emerging Technologies:

Technological advancements are merging with psychedelic therapy, fostering innovation:

- Virtual Reality (VR): Utilizing VR to enhance therapeutic experiences, create safe and immersive environments, and potentially reduce risks.
- Neurofeedback: Monitoring brain activity in real-time during psychedelic journeys to personalize interventions and optimize outcomes.
- Artificial Intelligence (AI): Leveraging AI to analyze data from research studies and individual therapeutic experiences to accelerate learning and personalize treatment plans.

Challenges and Opportunities:

Despite the vibrant landscape, challenges remain:

* Funding and Regulation: Securing funding for research and navigating complex regulatory hurdles continue to impede progress.
* Stigma and Misinformation: Countering stigma and addressing misinformation surrounding psychedelics is crucial for public acceptance and responsible integration.
* Accessibility and Equity: Ensuring equitable access to safe and effective psychedelic therapy for all, regardless of socioeconomic background, is paramount.

The Road Ahead:

The future of psychedelic therapy is filled with immense potential. By fostering collaboration between researchers, clinicians, policymakers, and the public, we can navigate the challenges, prioritize ethical considerations, and ensure this promising field blossoms into a valuable tool for healing and well-being.

Key Takeaways:

* Ongoing research is unlocking the secrets of how psychedelics work and refining therapeutic approaches.
* The field is expanding beyond traditional substances and exploring innovative technologies.
* Challenges remain, but the potential for positive impact is undeniable.

Join the Conversation:

- By engaging in informed dialogue, advocating for responsible research and equitable access, and supporting ethical practices, we can collectively shape a future where psychedelic therapy reaches its full potential and helps individuals and communities across the globe flourish.

- Remember, this book is for informational purposes only and is not a substitute for professional medical advice. Please consult with a qualified healthcare professional for guidance on mental health, treatment options, and navigating psychedelic experiences.

Chapter 14: Breaking the Stigma: Fostering Openness and Collaboration

As we stand at the precipice of a new era in mental health treatment with psychedelics, one crucial hurdle remains: stigma. Decades of misinformation, sensationalized media portrayals, and legal restrictions have cast a long shadow, hindering open dialogue, responsible research, and access to potential healing for those in need. This chapter delves into the importance of breaking the stigma surrounding psychedelics and fostering a collaborative approach to maximize their potential for positive impact.

From Forbidden to Open Dialogue:

For decades, psychedelics have been shrouded in secrecy, fear, and negative connotations. This stigma has:

- Discouraged individuals from seeking help: The fear of judgment and social stigma can prevent those who might benefit from psychedelic therapy from even considering it.
- Hindered research: Stigma has discouraged funding and participation in research, slowing down scientific exploration and progress.
- Fueled misinformation: The lack of open dialogue has created fertile ground for misinformation and sensationalized narratives, further perpetuating negative perceptions.

Breaking the Silence:

Shifting the narrative requires a multifaceted approach:

- Personal Stories: Sharing personal experiences of healing and positive transformation with psychedelics can challenge stereotypes and foster empathy.
- Education and Awareness: Raising awareness through accurate information, documentaries, and educational resources combats misinformation and promotes understanding.
- Open and Honest Dialogue: Engaging in open and honest dialogue about psychedelics, their potential benefits and risks, is crucial for destigmatization.
- Media Responsibility: Journalists and media outlets have a crucial role in portraying psychedelics responsibly, avoiding sensationalism and promoting evidence-based narratives.

Collaboration is Key:

Breaking down silos and fostering collaboration is essential:

- Researchers and Clinicians: Collaboration between researchers studying the mechanisms of action and clinicians providing therapeutic experiences can accelerate progress and ensure evidence-based practices.
- Policymakers and Public: Engaging policymakers in open dialogue about the potential of psychedelics and the need for responsible regulation can pave the way for wider access.
- Community and Advocacy Groups: Supporting community organizations and advocacy groups working to destigmatize psychedelics and promote responsible practices is vital.

A Shared Responsibility:

Breaking the stigma surrounding psychedelics is a shared
responsibility. By sharing personal stories, supporting educational
initiatives, engaging in open dialogue, and fostering collaboration,
we can create a more informed and accepting environment where
this promising field can reach its full potential for healing and
well-being.

Remember:

- Breaking stigma is an ongoing process that requires sustained
  effort and collaboration.
- Open and honest dialogue, based on facts and evidence, is
  crucial for overcoming misinformation and building trust.
- Sharing personal stories, while respecting individual privacy,
  can be a powerful tool for destigmatization and fostering
  empathy.
- By working together, we can create a future where psychedelics
  are seen not as taboo substances, but as valuable tools for
  healing and personal growth, accessible to those who can
  benefit most.
- This concludes our exploration of "The Shadow of Depression:
  A Beacon of Hope?". We hope this journey has informed,
  inspired, and empowered you to engage thoughtfully with the
  evolving field of psychedelic therapy and contribute to building
  a brighter future for mental health.

Chapter 15: Finding Your Path: Personalized Approaches to Mental Wellness

As we conclude this exploration of the potential of psychedelics for treating depression, it's crucial to remember that no single approach holds the universal key to unlocking mental well-being. This chapter emphasizes the importance of personalized journeys and highlights the diverse tools and practices available to support your unique path towards healing and growth.

Beyond the Psychedelic Horizon:

While psychedelics offer a glimmer of hope, they are not a magic bullet. Remember, mental well-being is a multifaceted journey shaped by various factors:

- Biological factors: Genetics, brain chemistry, and even gut health can influence mood and mental health.
- Psychological factors: Our thoughts, beliefs, coping mechanisms, and past experiences play a significant role.
- Social factors: Relationships, social support, and cultural influences significantly impact well-being.
- Lifestyle factors: Physical activity, sleep hygiene, diet, and substance use all contribute to mental health.

Embrace the Spectrum of Options:

Recognizing the diverse factors influencing mental well-being opens doors to a spectrum of potential approaches. Consider exploring:

- Therapy: Working with a qualified therapist can provide invaluable support, guidance, and tools to navigate emotional challenges, develop healthy coping mechanisms, and cultivate self-compassion.
- Mindfulness and Meditation: These practices can enhance self-awareness, emotional regulation, and present-moment focus, fostering inner peace and resilience.
- Lifestyle Changes: Prioritizing healthy sleep, regular physical activity, a balanced diet, and reducing stress can significantly improve mood and well-being.
- Community and Support Groups: Connecting with others who share similar experiences can provide a sense of belonging, understanding, and valuable social support.
- Creative Expression: Engaging in activities like art, music, writing, or movement can offer healthy outlets for processing emotions and fostering personal growth.
- Nature Connection: Spending time in nature has been shown to reduce stress, improve mood, and boost overall well-being.

Finding Your Unique Blend:

The most effective approach is often a personalized blend of these and other practices tailored to your individual needs and preferences. Experiment, explore, and find what resonates with you. Remember, there's no one-size-fits-all solution, and your journey is unique.

The Role of Psychedelics:

If you're considering incorporating psychedelics into your journey, approach them with informed awareness and responsible caution:

- Seek professional guidance: Consult with qualified healthcare professionals experienced in psychedelic therapy to ensure safety, suitability, and integration support.
- Prioritize ethical considerations: Ensure you are participating in legal and ethically sound practices.
- Integrate with intention: Don't view psychedelics as a quick fix, but as a potential catalyst for deeper healing and personal transformation. Integrate insights gained into your ongoing journey of well-being.

Remember:

You are not alone. Many individuals are exploring diverse paths to mental well-being, and support is available.

Be patient and compassionate with yourself. Healing is a journey, not a destination.
Celebrate your progress, no matter how small. Every step towards well-being is a step in the right direction.

Conclusion:

This exploration of "The Shadow of Depression: A Beacon of Hope?" has delved into the complex landscape of depression, the potential of psychedelics, and the importance of personalized approaches to mental well-being. As you move forward on your unique path, remember that hope exists, support is available, and you have the power to cultivate inner peace and well-being.

Disclaimer:

This book is for informational purposes only and is not a substitute for professional medical advice. Please consult with a qualified healthcare professional for guidance on mental health, treatment options, and navigating psychedelic experiences.

Chapter 16: Resources and Support: Connecting with Professionals and Communities

As you embark on your journey towards mental well-being, it's crucial to remember that you don't have to walk this path alone. A wealth of resources and supportive communities are available to guide and empower you. This chapter equips you with valuable tools to connect with qualified professionals and engage with supportive communities, fostering your path towards healing and growth.

Seeking Professional Guidance:

Finding the right mental health professional can be daunting, but it's an essential step in receiving personalized support and navigating your unique needs. Here are some resources to help you connect with qualified professionals:

- National Alliance on Mental Illness (NAMI): NAMI provides a helpline, support groups, and a wealth of resources to connect you with mental health professionals in your area. Visit their website at https://www.nami.org/.
- MentalHealth.gov: This government website offers a treatment locator tool to help you find mental health professionals in your area based on your insurance, location, and specific needs. Visit their website at https://www.mentalhealth.gov/.
- Psychology Today: This online directory allows you to search for therapists and counsellors based on their location, specialty, insurance acceptance, and other criteria. Visit their website at https://www.psychologytoday.com/us.
- American Psychological Association (APA): The APA offers a psychologist locator tool to help you find licensed psychologists in your area.

Considerations When Choosing a Therapist:

- **Qualifications:** Ensure the professional is licensed and holds relevant credentials in their field.
- **Experience:** Look for someone with experience treating individuals with similar challenges or concerns.
- **Therapeutic Approach:** Choose a therapist whose approach aligns with your preferences and needs.
- **Personality and Comfort Level:** Feeling comfortable and safe with your therapist is crucial for open communication and effective treatment.
- **Gut Feeling:** never ignore any an easiness you fell when you meet a Therapist. Always go with your gut, it can save your mind and your money.

Exploring Psychedelic Therapy:

If you're considering exploring psychedelic therapy, approaching it with informed awareness and responsible caution is paramount. Here are some resources to help you navigate this path:

- MAPS (Multidisciplinary Association for Psychedelic Studies): MAPS conducts research and advocacy for the therapeutic use of psychedelics. Visit their website at [invalid URL removed].
- Heffter Research Institute: This institute conducts research on the therapeutic potential of psilocybin and other psychedelics. Visit their website at https://www.heffter.org/.
- Fireside Project: This organization provides resources and support for individuals seeking psychedelic therapy experiences. Visit their website at https://firesideproject.org/.

Remember:

- Seek professional guidance: Consult with qualified healthcare professionals experienced in psychedelic therapy to ensure safety, suitability, and integration support.
- Prioritize ethical considerations: Ensure you are participating in legal and ethically sound practices.
- Integrate with intention: Don't view psychedelics as a quick fix, but as a potential catalyst for deeper healing and personal transformation.

Finding Your Community:

Connecting with others who share similar experiences can provide invaluable support, understanding, and a sense of belonging. Here are some communities you can explore:

- NAMI Support Groups: NAMI offers a network of support groups for individuals and families affected by mental illness. Visit their website to find a group near you: https://www.nami.org/Support-Education/Support-Groups.
- MentalHealth.gov Online Communities: This website offers online communities where you can connect with others who are struggling with mental health challenges.
- Psychedelic Therapy Communities: Several online communities and forums exist for individuals interested in exploring psychedelic therapy. However, it's crucial to approach these communities with caution and discernment, prioritizing reliable sources and information.

Remember:

- Engage critically: Evaluate the information and advice shared in online communities with a critical eye and consult with qualified professionals for guidance.
- Choose supportive spaces: Seek communities that foster respectful dialogue, avoid misinformation, and prioritize ethical practices.
- Protect your privacy: Be mindful of what personal information you share online and prioritize your safety and well-being.

Conclusion

A Message of Hope: Embracing the Potential of Psychedelics for a Brighter Future

As we reach the culmination of this exploration, a beacon of hope shines brightly. The potential of psychedelics for treating depression and other mental health challenges offers a transformative glimpse into a future where healing and well-being are more accessible than ever before.

This journey has delved into the complexities of depression, the fascinating science behind psychedelics, and the diverse tapestry of personal stories that illuminate their potential. We have explored the ethical considerations, legal landscape, and the importance of responsible exploration.

While challenges remain, the momentum is undeniable. Research is flourishing, public perception is shifting, and communities are coming together to advocate for responsible access and ethical practices.

Remember:
- Hope exists: Don't let the shadow of depression obscure the light of hope. There are effective treatments available, and psychedelics offer a promising new frontier.
- You are not alone: Millions of individuals around the world struggle with mental health challenges. Support systems, communities, and qualified professionals are here to walk alongside you.
- Be your own advocate: Educate yourself, explore your options, and make informed decisions about your well-being.
- Seek guidance from qualified professionals and prioritize your safety and well-being.

Call to Action: Joining the Conversation and Advocating for Change

The future of mental health is in our hands. We can all play a role in shaping a brighter tomorrow by:

- Engaging in open and honest dialogue: Share your experiences, challenge stigma, and promote understanding about mental health and psychedelics.
- Supporting research and advocacy: Donate to organizations conducting responsible research and advocating for ethical access to psychedelic therapy.
- Prioritizing ethical considerations: Advocate for responsible regulations, support legal frameworks that prioritize safety and well-being, and hold practitioners accountable to ethical standards.
- Creating supportive communities: Foster safe spaces where individuals can share their experiences, find support, and connect with others on their journeys towards healing.

Together, we can:

- Destigmatize mental health and create a world where seeking help is seen as a sign of strength, not weakness.
- Ensure equitable access to safe and effective mental health treatments, including responsible forms of psychedelic therapy.
- Empower individuals to take ownership of their well-being and cultivate a future where mental health flourishes for all.
- Remember, you are a powerful force for change. Embrace the potential within yourself and join the movement towards a brighter future for mental health.

This concludes our exploration of "The Shadow of Depression: A Beacon of Hope?". We hope this journey has empowered you to engage thoughtfully with the evolving field of psychedelic therapy and contribute to building a world where well-being thrives.

Disclaimer:

This book is for informational purposes only and is not a substitute for professional medical advice. Please consult with a qualified healthcare professional for guidance on mental health, treatment options, and navigating psychedelic experiences.

A Call to Action:

As we conclude this journey, remember that the conversation doesn't end here. We must continue to engage in responsible research, open dialogue, and advocacy to ensure the potential of this field is harnessed ethically and effectively. Together, we can navigate this path with hope, caution, and a shared commitment to building a brighter future for mental health.

Thank you for joining us on this exploration of the psychedelic frontier. May this journey inspire you to learn more, engage thoughtfully, and advocate for a future where access to safe and effective mental health interventions is a reality for all.

We hope this journey has informed, inspired, and empowered you to engage thoughtfully with this evolving field and contribute to building a brighter future for mental health.

Case studies

Real Stories of Transformation: Personal Accounts of Healing with Psychedelics
Disclaimer: The following stories are based on real experiences but have been modified to protect individual privacy. Please consult with a qualified healthcare professional before considering any form of self-treatment.

Story 1: **Sarah's Journey with Psilocybin**

Sarah had battled crippling depression for years. Traditional medications offered little relief, leaving her feeling numb and disconnected. As a last resort, she enrolled in a psilocybin-assisted therapy program. Under the guidance of a trained therapist, Sarah embarked on a series of journeys that unfolded like vibrant dreamscapes. She confronted past traumas, experienced overwhelming love and acceptance, and gained a newfound appreciation for life's beauty. "Psilocybin wasn't a magic bullet," Sarah reflects, "but it cracked open a door I didn't know existed. It allowed me to revisit my pain, understand its roots, and finally let go." Today, Sarah lives a fulfilling life, managing her depression with therapy and mindfulness practices learned through her psychedelic experience.

Story 2: **Mark's Breakthrough with Ketamine**

Mark, a veteran haunted by PTSD, felt constantly on edge, burdened by nightmares and flashbacks. Ketamine-assisted therapy offered a glimmer of hope. During his sessions, Mark relived traumatic memories in a controlled setting, experiencing them with newfound compassion and understanding. The emotional intensity helped him release the grip of fear and begin to forgive himself. "Ketamine didn't erase my past," Mark shares, "but it helped me rewrite the narrative. Now, I can access memories without being overwhelmed, and that's made a world of difference."

Story 3: **Emily's Discovery of Self-Compassion with MDMA**

Emily struggled with debilitating social anxiety, feeling isolated and trapped within her own fears. MDMA-assisted therapy provided a safe space for introspection and connection. The therapy sessions fostered deep self-compassion as Emily explored her anxieties and vulnerabilities. "MDMA opened my heart," Emily explains, "it allowed me to see myself with kindness and understanding. Now, I have the courage to connect with others and build meaningful relationships."

Story 4: **David's Healing Transformation with Mindfulness**

David suffered from chronic anxiety that manifested as constant worry and physical tension. Medication offered temporary relief, but he yearned for a deeper solution. He discovered mindfulness meditation, practicing techniques like focused breathing and body awareness. With regular practice, David learned to calm his racing mind, cultivate inner peace, and manage his anxiety without medication. "Mindfulness wasn't easy," David admits, "but the payoff has been immense. I now have tools to manage my anxiety and live a more present and peaceful life."

A Beacon of Hope

These personal stories offer a glimpse into the diverse ways individuals have found healing through psychedelic therapy and alternative approaches. Remember, everyone's journey is unique. If you are struggling with mental health challenges, please reach out to a qualified professional to explore safe and effective treatment options. There is hope, and your path to healing awaits.

Self-Assessment Tools for Mental Well-being

Free Online Assessments:

Depression and Anxiety Screening Tests:
Beck Depression Inventory (BDI):
https://www.ismanet.org/doctoryourspirit/pdfs/Beck-Depression-Inventory-BDI.pdf

Generalized Anxiety Disorder 7-Item Scale (GAD-7):
https://www.nimh.nih.gov/health/trials/generalized-anxiety-disorder
Patient Health Questionnaire (PHQ-9):
https://www.phqscreeners.com/

Mindfulness and Stress Assessments:
Mindfulness Attention Awareness Scale (MAAS):
https://ggsc.berkeley.edu/images/uploads/The_Mindful_Attention_Awareness_Scale_-_Trait_(1).pdf

Perceived Stress Scale (PSS): https://psycnet.apa.org/getdoi.cfm?doi=10.1037/t02889-000

Overall Well-being Assessments:
World Health Organization (WHO) Well-being Index:
https://ogg.osu.edu/media/documents/MB%20Stream/who5.pdf

Five Factor Well-being Scale (FFWS):
https://www.hsph.harvard.edu/health-happiness/research-new/positive-health/measurement-of-well-being/

Mobile Apps:

Headspace: Guided meditations and mindfulness exercises
Calm: Soothing soundscapes and sleep stories
Happify: Interactive activities and games based on positive psychology
Insight Timer: Large community for meditation and mindfulness practice
Moodtrack: Track your mood and identify triggers

Additional Resources:

National Institute of Mental Health: https://www.nimh.nih.gov/
MentalHealth.gov: https://www.samhsa.gov/mental-health
The Jed Foundation: https://jedfoundation.org/
The Trevor Project: https://www.thetrevorproject.org/
National Suicide Prevention Lifeline: 988 (US)
Beckley Foundation: https://beckleyfoundation.org
Fireside Project: https://firesideproject.org
Heffter Research Institute: https:// Heffter.org
National Alliance on Mental Illness (NAMI): https://www.nami.org/
MentalHealth.gov: https://www.mentalhealth.gov/
Erowid.org (Use with caution and critical thinking):

Crisis Hotlines:
National Suicide Prevention Lifeline: 988 (US)
Crisis Text Line: Text HOME to 741741 (US)
The Trevor Project: 1-866-488-7386 (US)
Trans Lifeline: 1-877-565-8860 (US)

Mental Health Organizations:

National Alliance on Mental Illness (NAMI):
https://www.nami.org/
MentalHealth.gov: https://www.mentalhealth.gov/
The Jed Foundation: https://jedfoundation.org/
The Trevor Project: https://www.thetrevorproject.org/
American Foundation for Suicide Prevention (AFSP):
https://afsp.org/
National Suicide Prevention Lifeline:
https://suicidepreventionlifeline.org/
National Alliance on Mental Illness (NAMI)
Depression and Bipolar Support Alliance (DBSA)
Anxiety and Depression Association of America (ADAA):

Finding Qualified Professionals:

The Jed Foundation
Psychology Today:
https://www.psychologytoday.com/us/therapists
American Psychological Association (APA)
National Association of Social Workers (NASW)
MentalHealth.gov: https://www.mentalhealth.gov/
National Institute of Mental Health (NIMH):

Note: URLs links and phone numbers change without notice, this is the information available during the writing of this book. So i opted to give you the names of the organizations so you might easily google them, if you so find that a URL links are no longer working.

Disclaimer:

This book is for informational purposes only and is not intended
as a substitute for professional medical advice. Please consult
with a qualified healthcare professional before making any
decisions regarding your mental health or treatment options. All
resources in this book are to be explored by the reader and are not
a personal endorsement from the author, neither are they affiliate
links. Make informed decisions.

Remember:

Self-assessment tools are not a substitute for professional
diagnosis or treatment.
If you are experiencing significant mental health challenges,
please reach out to a qualified healthcare professional.
**These resources are a starting point for self-awareness and
exploration.**

Keep in mind the importance of self-compassion and seeking
professional help when needed.

I hope this helps.

Please remember that you are not alone.

Appendix: Glossary of Terms

Part 1: Demystifying Depression

Glossary of Key Terms:

Part 1: The Darkness Within

Depression: A common and debilitating mood disorder characterized by persistent sadness, loss of interest or pleasure, and other symptoms that significantly impair daily life.
Serotonin: A neurotransmitter that plays a role in mood, sleep, appetite, and other functions.
Norepinephrine: A neurotransmitter involved in alertness, mood, and focus.
Dopamine: A neurotransmitter associated with pleasure, reward, and motivation.
Neurotransmitters: Chemical messengers in the brain that transmit signals between nerve cells.
Neurons: Nerve cells that transmit information throughout the brain and body.
Hippocampus: A brain region involved in memory and learning.
Amygdala: A brain region responsible for processing emotions, particularly fear and anxiety.
Prefrontal cortex: The area of the brain responsible for executive functions like planning, decision-making, and self-control.
Genetics: The study of genes and their role in heredity.
Genetic predisposition: An increased likelihood of developing a certain condition due to inherited genes.
Epigenetics: The study of how environmental factors can influence gene expression without altering the DNA sequence itself.
Mental health: A state of well-being in which an individual realizes his or her own abilities, can cope with the normal stresses

of life, can work productively and fruitfully, and is able to make a contribution to his or her community.

Part 2: A Glimpse into the Light

Psychedelics: A class of drugs that produce profound changes in perception, mood, and cognition.
Psychedelic therapy: A form of therapy that uses psychedelics in a controlled setting to treat mental health conditions.
Psilocybin: A naturally occurring psychedelic compound found in certain mushrooms.
MDMA (Ecstasy): A synthetic psychedelic drug with stimulant and empathogenic properties.
Ayahuasca: A brew containing DMT, a naturally occurring psychedelic compound, and other psychoactive plants.
Ibogaine: A naturally occurring psychedelic compound found in the iboga plant.
Set and Setting: The internal and external environment in which a psychedelic experience takes place, both significantly impacting the experience itself.
Microdosing: Taking very low doses of psychedelics, often regularly, for potential benefits such as enhanced creativity and well-being.
Mechanism of action: The specific biological processes through which a drug produces its effects.
Neuroplasticity: The brain's ability to change and adapt throughout life.
Ego dissolution: A temporary loss of the sense of self that can occur during a psychedelic experience.
Mystical experience: A profound feeling of connection to something larger than oneself, often reported during psychedelic journeys.
Integration: The process of reflecting on and incorporating the insights gained from a psychedelic experience into daily life.

Part 3: Beyond the Horizon

Stigma: A negative association with a person or group, often based on prejudice or misconception.
Accessibility: The ability for individuals to access and afford healthcare, including psychedelic therapy.
Regulation: The establishment of laws and guidelines to govern the use of psychedelics.
Clinical trials: Research studies designed to assess the safety and efficacy of new treatments.
Phase I, II, and III trials: Different stages of clinical trials with increasing numbers of participants and complexity.
Double-blind study: A research design where neither participants nor researchers know who is receiving the active drug or a placebo.
Anecdotal evidence: Personal stories or experiences, not considered scientific evidence.
Placebo: A substance or treatment that is identical to the active drug in appearance but has no therapeutic effect.
Open-label study: A research design where participants and researchers know who is receiving the active drug or a placebo.
Naturalistic study: Research conducted in real-world settings, observing how treatments are used in everyday practice.
Meta-analysis: A statistical method that combines the results of multiple studies to draw more robust conclusions.
Informed consent: The process of providing individuals with all the necessary information about a treatment before they agree to participate.
Harm reduction: Strategies aimed at minimizing the risks associated with drug use.
Harm potential: The potential for a drug to cause adverse effects.
Addiction: A chronic, relapsing brain disease characterized by compulsive drug seeking and use, despite negative consequences.

Additional Terms:

HTR2A receptor: A serotonin receptor implicated in the effects of psychedelics like psilocybin and LSD.
5HTTLPR gene: A gene associated with serotonin regulation and potentially linked to depression and

Disclaimer: This glossary is not intended to be a substitute for professional medical advice. Consult a qualified healthcare professional for diagnosis and treatment of mental health conditions.